My NICU Story

Written with Love

#1 International Best Seller

Tiffani Jean Freckleton, RN, NTMC

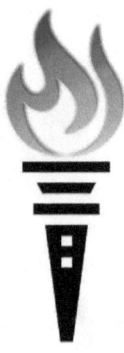

My NICU Story
Written With Love

Copyright © 2022 by Tiffani Jean Freckleton

Illustrations by Nicholas R. Massarella

Inspired Legacy Publishing is a division of (DBA) Inspired Legacy, LLC
PO Box 900816
Sandy UT 84090-0816

All rights reserved. No part of this publication may be reproduced distributed or transmitted in any form or by any means including photocopying recording or other electronic or mechanical means without proper written permission of author or publisher, except in the case of brief quotations embodied in critical reviews and certain other noncommercial uses permitted by copyright law.

ISBN 979-8-9866355-0-7 (paperback)
ISBN 979-8-9866355-1-4 (hardcover)

Printed in the United States of America

What People Are Saying

"Ms. Tiffani Freckleton shares with her readers a warm and loving perspective of a newborn cared for in the Neonatal Intensive Care Unit (NICU)."
—Wendy K. Benson, MBA, OTR/L and Elizabeth A. Myers, RN
Co-authors, The Confident Patient, 2x2 Health: Private Health Concierge

"A must read for anyone who is on or has been through a NICU journey."
—Tyra Wright, NICU mom of a 34-week preemie

"This book helped me feel seen as a NICU parent...Highly recommend!"
—Heather Williams, NICU mom of a 31-week preemie

"Parents who have babies in the NICU are experiencing all types of emotions, so it was heartwarming to read something from a different perspective. Well written!"
—Wendy L. Hooton, NICU mom, Down Syndrome Advocate, Author

"My NICU Story is a beautifully written journey as told from an infant's point of view. I would highly recommend this book to anyone walking through the NICU doors."
—Krista Burrow Nuttall, Speech-language Pathologist, Neonatal Therapist

Dedicated to all mothers and fathers; adoptive, birth, and foster.

And to my own parents,
Douglas & Lauren

Dear NICU parent,

Congratulations on the birth of your child!

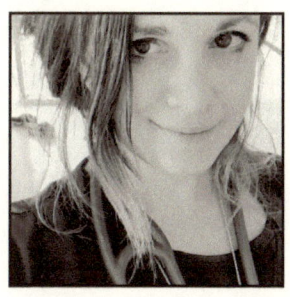

Welcome to the Neonatal Intensive Care Unit, more affectionately known as the NICU. This is a special place in the hospital for the tiniest of patients. You and your baby are in wonderful hands here. Each baby comes to the NICU for different reasons and every experience is unique. Whether you are counting down the days, or counting down the weeks; there is good in every day, although some days you might have to search a little harder.

I love the phrase, "Every baby tells their own story." Because without a doubt, your infant is the one in charge. Babies are so smart, and they know how to guide you along the way. Softer than a whisper, you just have to listen close. There are no illustrations in this book because the NICU stay is different for each and every one of you. I honor your story.

My wish is to bring you some comfort in this difficult time. I know it's hard. I know this wasn't your plan. It's not your fault. When I became a nurse in the NICU I was overcome by the love, and each baby's individual special personality. I have seen how powerful your voice is. I hope you will read this book aloud. That it might help you bond with your sweet infant. Trust me, you are doing enough. Your voice, your touch, your love is magic.

I have found that sometimes in the most unexpected, dark places, there is still light; you can find joy you never knew existed. You are strong enough.

From behind the scenes, inspired by NICU... you got this!

Tiffani RN

My NICU Story

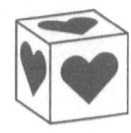

I'm a newborn baby in the I.C.U.
This is my story, from me to you.

NICU babies come in all different sizes.
Often, we arrive with a few surprises.

But,

We each write our story in our very own way.
So let's try to take it day by day.

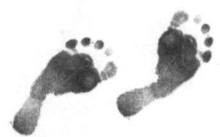

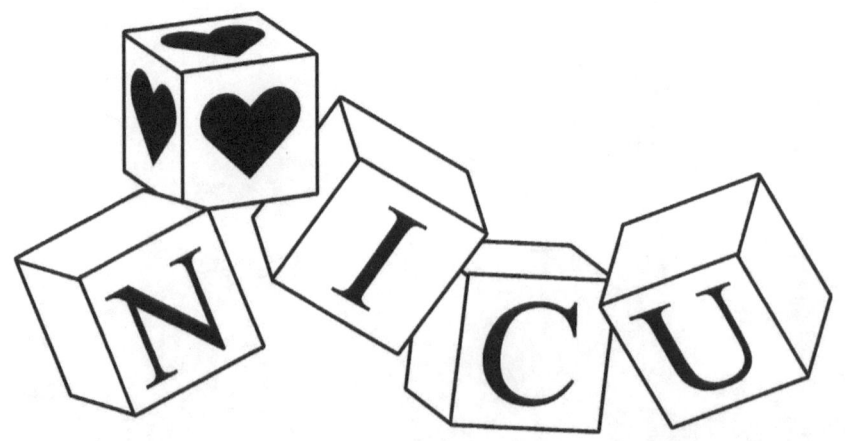

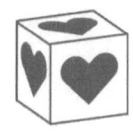

I promise the NICU is a special place to be.
Maybe it's scary for you, it feels safe to me.

Please don't forget that you're not alone.
There's so much help 'til I come home.

Swaddle me tight, tuck my arms and legs inside.
Some days might feel like a roller coaster ride.

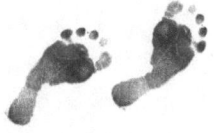

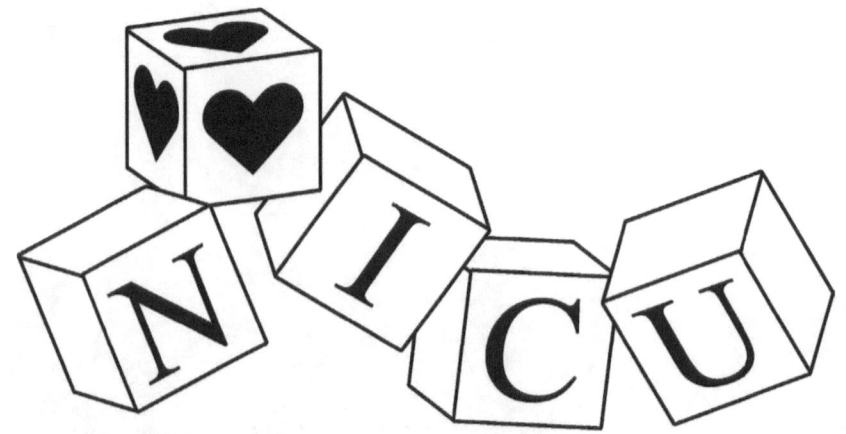

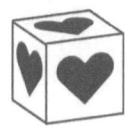

The ups and downs will come and go.
But I'm so much stronger than you know.

My sweet parent, I see you.
Thanks for all of the things you do.

Enjoy this journey along the way.
Our time together, a treasure each day.

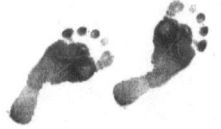

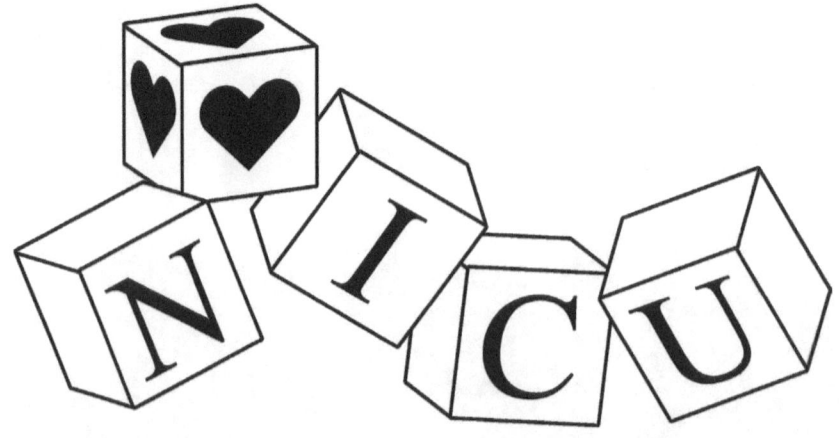

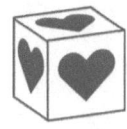

And just like me, my goals are so small.
Embrace the good and celebrate them all.

Talk to me softly, place your finger in my hand.
These are things I understand.

I know your voice, and oh, I love your touch.
Trust me, I know, you're doing enough.

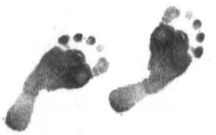

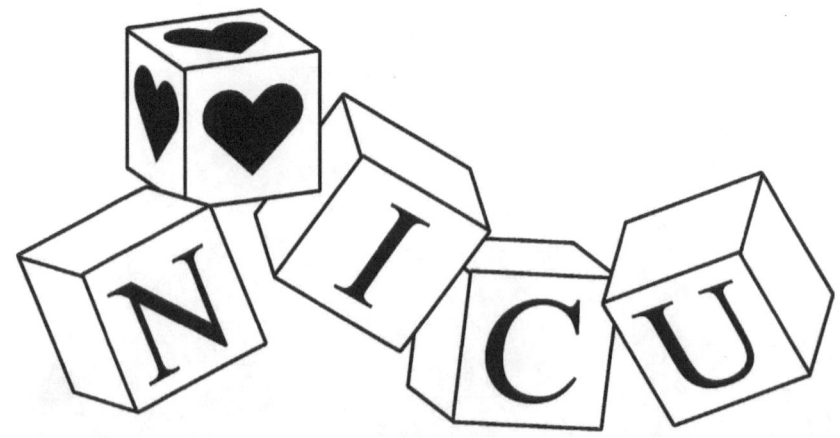

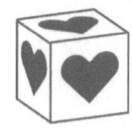

I love how you wrap me sweetly, nice, and snug.

It comforts me, as your hands give hugs.

We get special times no one tells you about.

The littlest of things are what really count.

Remember that moment, when you held me first.

Our hearts so full of love, about to burst.

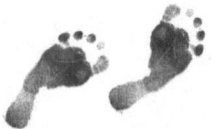

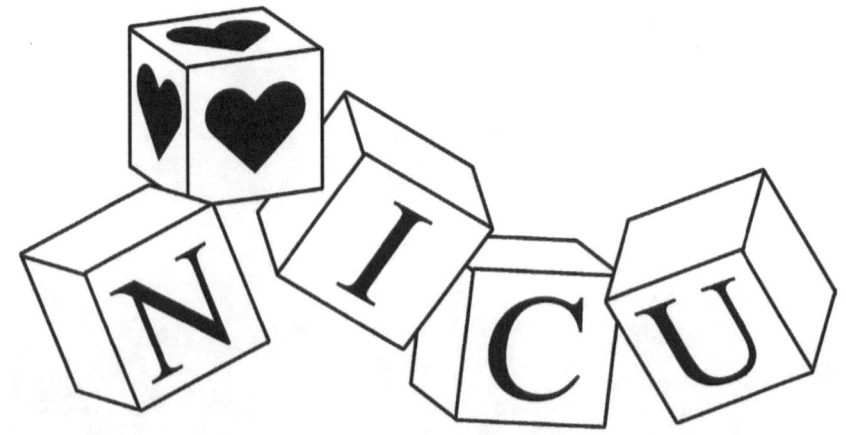

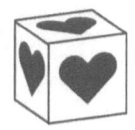

Holding me close, against your chest.
Hearing your heartbeat, it's the best.

As I start to wear clothes, when you give me a bath,
the milestones add up, just do the math.

I know some days, it feels really tough.
I'll tell you again, you're doing enough.

You give me strength to do my best,
allowing my little body time to rest.

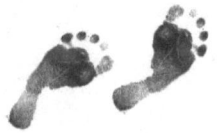

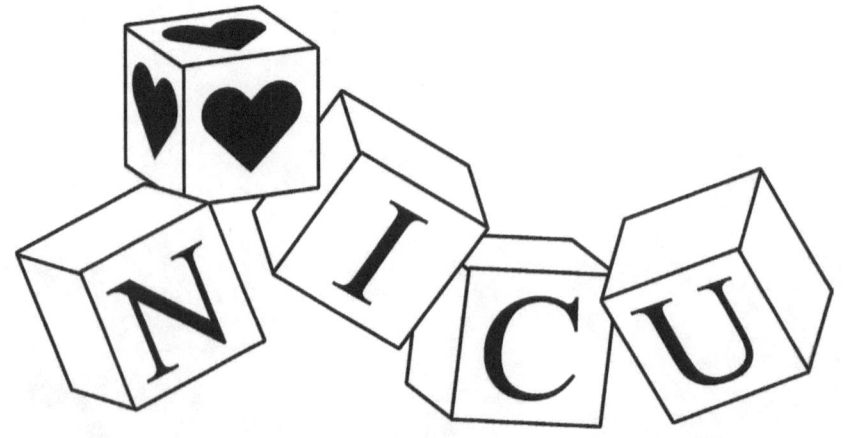

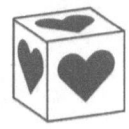

You'll see every few hours my schedule goes;
Sleep, eat, and repeat! While I grow.

I'm learning to eat at my own pace.
I hear it's a marathon, and not a race.

I'll let you know when it's time to stop.
When I don't even want one more drop.

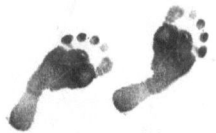

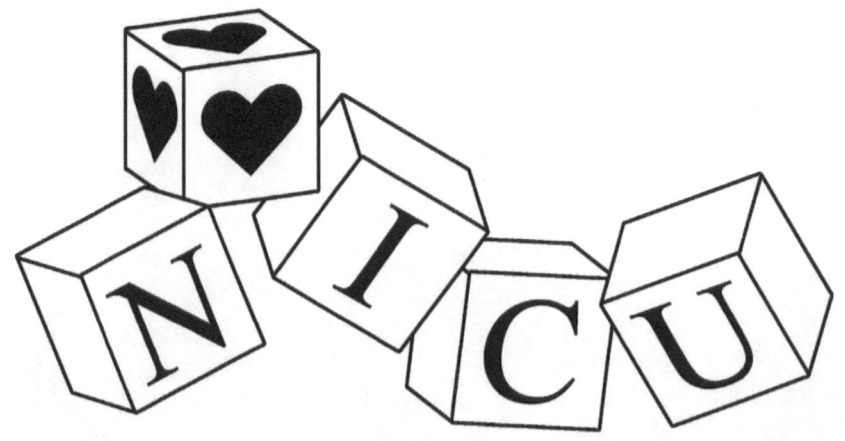

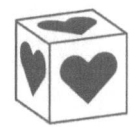

It's so much work learning new things.
It doesn't bother me, when I hear alarms ring.

Everyone here, knows just what to do.
They keep me safe, until I can be with you.

Please take a deep breath, and so will I.
Go ahead, when you need to cry.

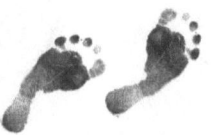

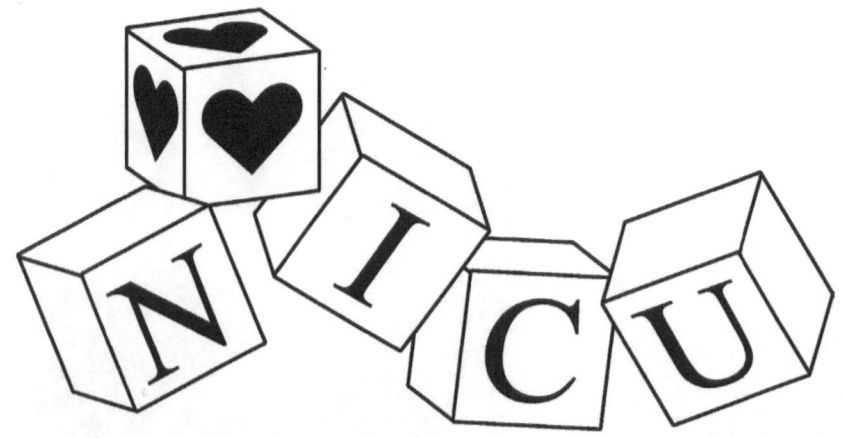

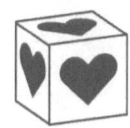

After the tears, a rainbow appears.
Think of me, and ease some of those fears.

I know it's the worst, as you're driving home.
How it feels you're leaving me all alone.

But just like angels from up above,
I promise,
I'm surrounded by so much love.

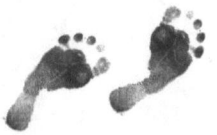

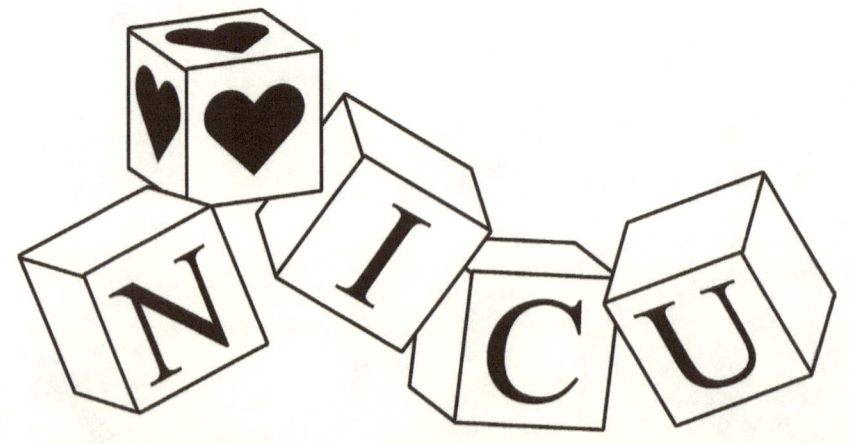

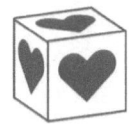

Honestly, it's a blessing in disguise,
getting to know these NICU guys.

I hear them walking through my door.
Oohing and aahing, they stop to adore.

Giving whispers of hope, smiles of joy.
To all of us babes, each girl and boy.

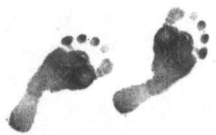

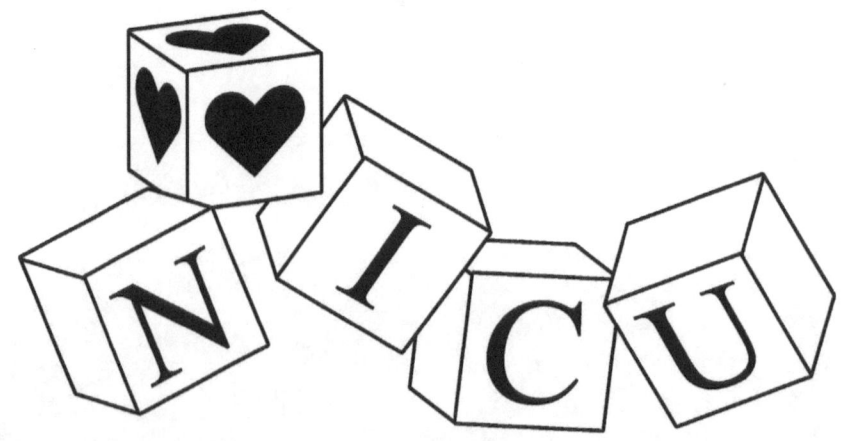

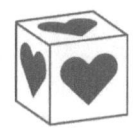

Then, suddenly that happy day is here.
We shout hooray and all will cheer!

I'm coming home! We made it through.
But there's one more thing I need from you.

Thank the NICU from me,
when it's time for good-byes.
For helping you out, for silencing my cries.

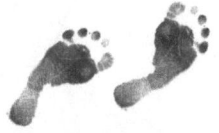

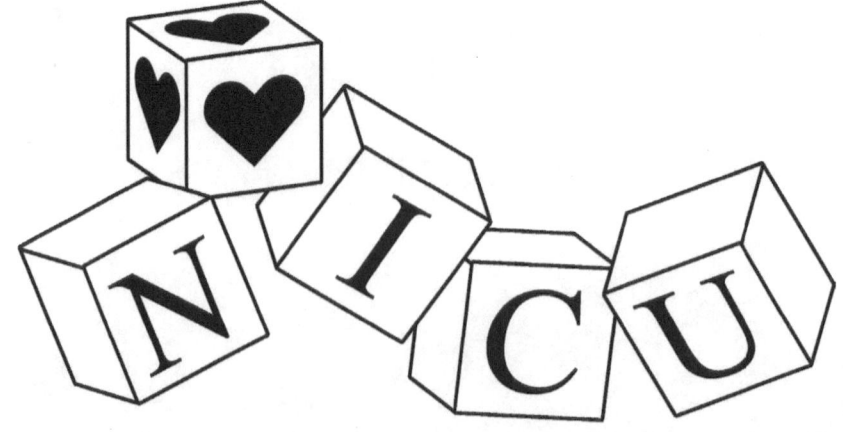

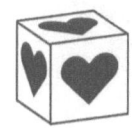

All of their hearts have helped me grow,
into the strong baby, that you now know.

When you walk out the doors for the very last time,
is your heart beating as fast as mine?

Down the long hallway, each step held by you.
Going home at last, our dreams come true.

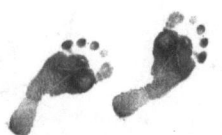

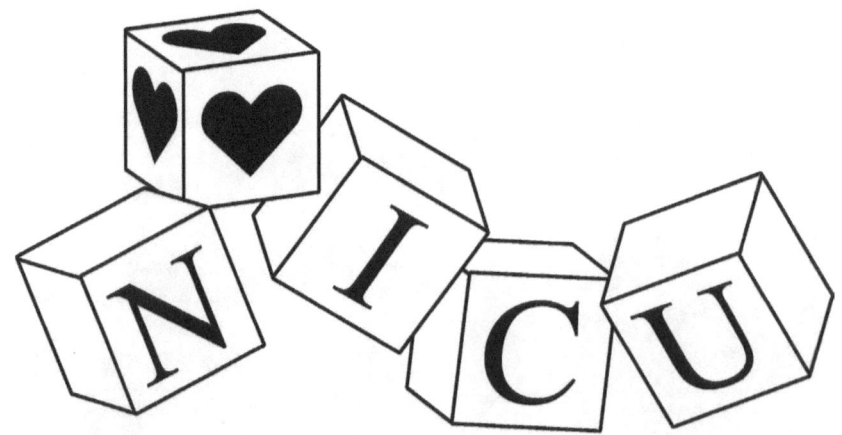

♥ Final Thoughts →

I'm just a nurse in the N.I.C.U.
This is my story from me to you.

The NICU is a special place to be,
and sometimes it's even scary for me.

I'm trying my best to do enough,
I had no idea it would be so tough.

I want so much to ease your fears,
I see your worry, my eyes fill with tears.

Your baby is loved, more than you know.
I got your back after you go.

Oh, I love their stories, and I know their names.
I promise you, no baby's the same.

It's an honor to care for your babe,
helping you find the good in each day.

Now, there's only one thing left to do...

From my heart to yours;
thank you for allowing me be a part of your story.

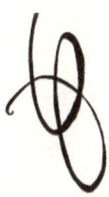

About the Author

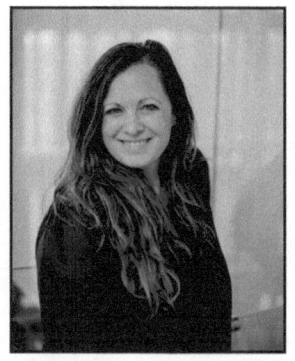

Tiffani Jean Freckleton graduated from Dixie State College of Utah in 2004. After many years as a registered nurse, she discovered what she believes is the best kept secret in healthcare: the Neonatal Intensive Care Unit, aka the NICU. Tiffani is certified in Neonatal Touch and Massage (NTMC) and loves her NICU babes.

As a nurse, her perspective of the NICU is from behind the scenes. She has been deeply inspired by the NICU, and all of the precious baby's stories.

She is the aunt to seven nephews and one niece, four of whom are NICU graduates, each with their own unique story. Tiffani's first love is reading. She only recently discovered she likes writing as well. She adores football, attempts yoga, tries her best to cook, and enjoys the idea of having a garden.

My contact info:

Instagram: @just_tiffer
            @bookstagramandread
            @inspiredbynicu

Email: tiff.freck@outlook.com

Nephew #1

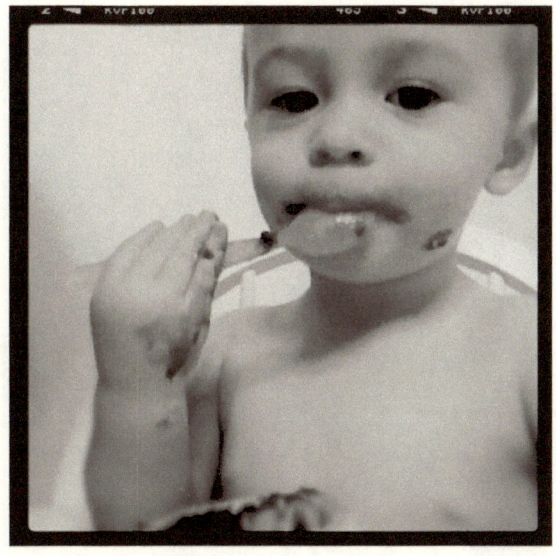

Nephew #1- January 2011. ♥ "I will show my Aunt Tiff unconditional love"

This kid. He has gifted me with a special kind of unconditional love. I didn't get kids of my own. Yet, he has always made enough love in his heart for me as if he was a little bit part mine. My first Instagram post of him came from our Mondays together. (The only day of the week his parents schedule overlapped, I would babysit him every Monday). Although he was not the first reason why I love being an aunt, he easily became the best thing about it.

Nephew #2

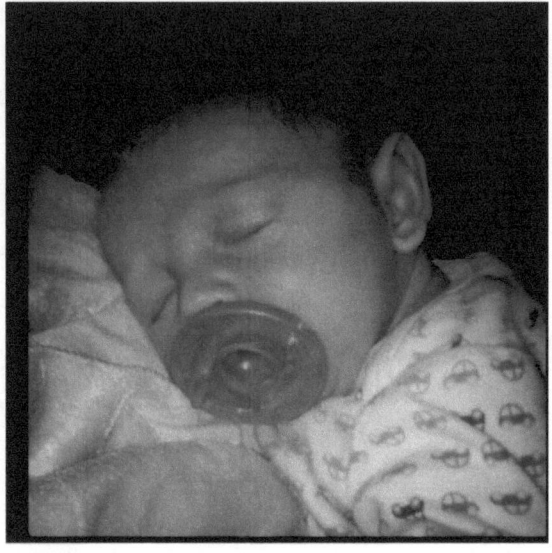

Nephew #2- November 2014 💟 "I will teach my Aunt Tiff how to be brave"

This is the most fearless kid I know. My second nephew, full of love and full of trouble. His older brother loved me, so he did too. Trust me when I say being an aunt is the easy job! This is when I started making photo books for my nephews. The perfect mix of his parents and still the coolest kid I know.

♡ Nephew #3 →

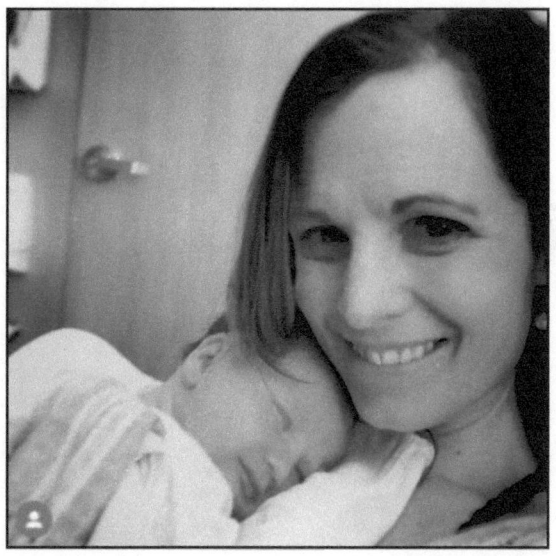

Nephew #3- April 2015 💜 *"I'll be my Aunt Tiff's friend when she needs one the most"*

So ready and so in love with this guy joining our family. The first born of his family gets a special place in my heart, (since I'm the first born in mine).
He was my best friend when I needed one the most. Babysitting him helped heal my broken heart after my divorce. This is when I read the book that changed my life. This is when I created my best photo albums for my nephews.

Nephew #4

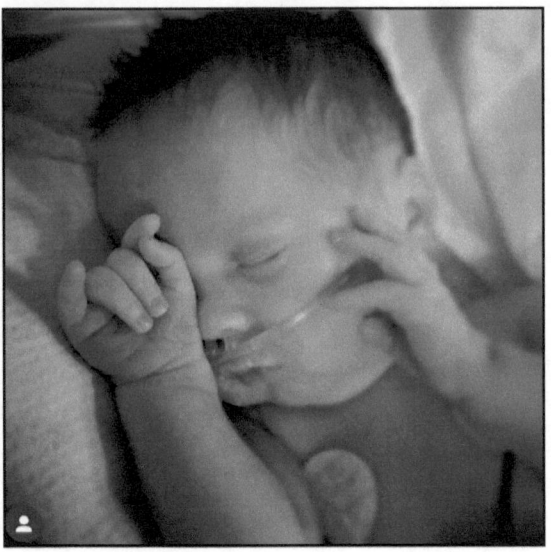

Nephew #4 February 2016 🖤 *"I'll teach my Aunt Tiff about the NICU"*

Not even a year after his brother, this guy showed up at 31 weeks. My first real experience with the NICU, despite being a nurse for over ten years. I couldn't believe how much these nurses helped my brother and his wife. They would pick up his older brother from our adventures of babysitting with stories of how much the NICU nurses loved our feisty guy. "Can you believe he has a temper!" "How can a baby have a temper?" He did then, he does now. Who knew, only a NICU nurse.

Nephew #5

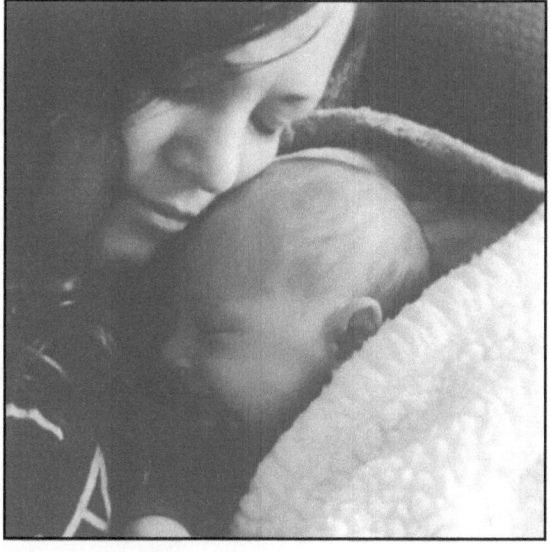

Nephew #5 January 2020 💜 "I'll remind my Aunt Tiff about the NICU"

Fast forward...A few years later, still full of questions about what to do with my life. This cute guy showed up with just a brief visit to the NICU. Every since his cousin before him, I've wondered whether that was the better path for me. He arrived as I was applying for new jobs, a NICU position was posted. The day I drove hours to meet him began with submitting my application to the NICU.

Nephew #6

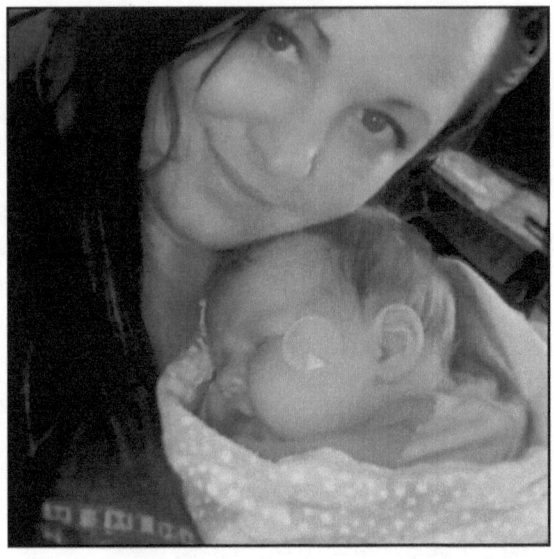

Nephew #6 July 2020 🩶 "I'll inspire my Aunt Tiff to write a book"

I did it. I started as a NICU nurse March 2020. The very week COVID changed the world as we knew it. A few months later this guy arrived in the NICU. But not in my hospital, and unable to even visit, I felt helpless. I hadn't made a photo book for my nephews since his brother was in the NICU years before. It was time to do something. Wanting to be a better aunt, sister, nurse... i thought of this guy every day. And I started writing.

Niece #1

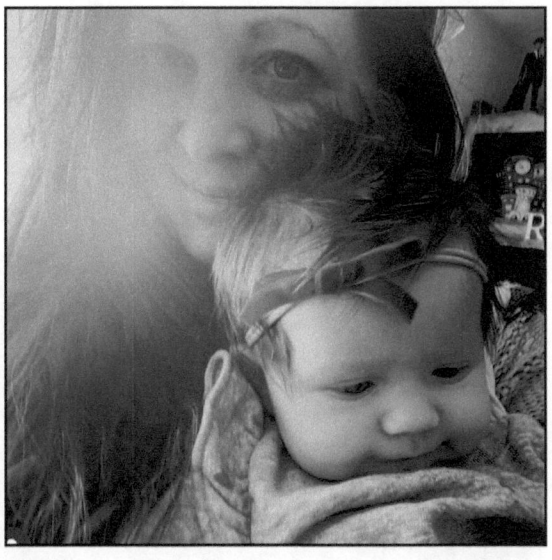

Finally, a niece! December 2021 💟 "I get to share my Aunt Tiff's middle name!"

I'm the oldest, with younger brothers. Who only had only boys, until now. Until her! And we get to share the same middle name. After her mother. And her great grandmother, but I'm there too. Unlike her older brothers, our Christmas miracle skipped the NICU altogether. By now we just started to expect the NICU, but little miss surprised us all.

Nephew #7

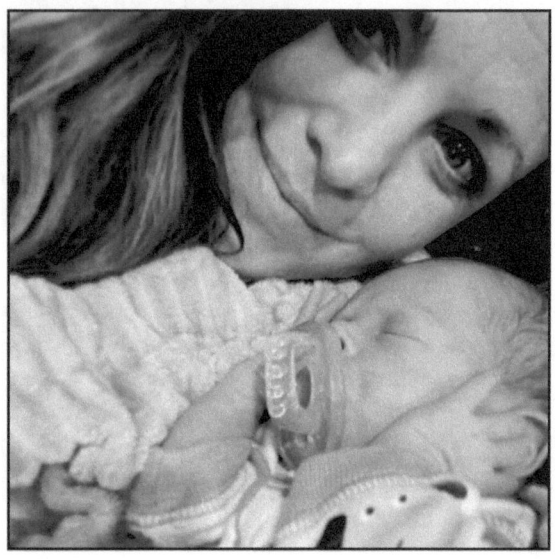

Nephew #7 March 2022 💚 "I got this!....aka.....I'll help my Aunt Tiff finish her book"

He showed up one day, with the drama only a baby can bring. Earlier than planned, in the NICU, not in the NICU, then back to the NICU again. I was preparing my book for beta readers, his cousin had skipped the NICU so my first draft was a gift to a different brother and his wife. This sassy pants even helped me with some last missing words. Even when you expect to be in the NICU, it won't be like you expect.

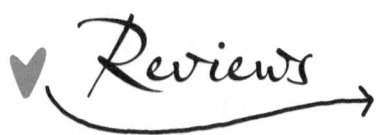

"Ms. Tiffani Freckleton shares with her readers a warm and loving perspective of a newborn cared for in the Neonatal Intensive Care Unit (NICU). Coming from a place of the deep understanding from a seasoned NICU nurse, the author gifts her patients and their parents with a compassionate and supportive message that can, and should be read aloud to their loved ones again and again!"
—Wendy K. Benson, MBA, OTR/L and Elizabeth A. Myers, RN
Co-authors, The Confident Patient, 2x2 Health: Private Health Concierge, http://www.2x2health.com/

"This story is a heartwarming gift to NICU parents. It captures the NICU experience so well from the sweetest perspective. A must read for anyone who is on or has been through a NICU journey."
—Tyra Wright, NICU mom of a 34-week preemie

"This book helped me feel seen as a NICU parent. It allowed me to recognize how hard my baby was fighting to be with me, rather than how hard we were all fighting against time and hospital hoops. Highly recommend!"
—Heather Williams, NICU mom of a 31-week preemie

"I enjoyed reading My NICU Story written by a nurse who provides care for babies who are in the NICU. Parents who have babies in the NICU are experiencing all types of emotions, so it was heartwarming to read something from a different perspective. I love the idea of a small being providing comfort to its parents at a time they feel they need to do everything for him/her. This book may possibly be just what these parents need. Well written!"
—Wendy L. Hooton, NICU mom, Down Syndrome Advocate, Author

"My NICU Story is a beautifully written journey as told from an infant's point of view. Poetically written, this story takes you down the path of experiences and emotions that a baby and their family encounter during their NICU stay.

Reading it I felt hopeful. As a NICU healthcare provider I appreciate the perspective it gave. I imagine parents, healthcare providers, friends, family and NICU babies who have grown into children reading it over and over again to experience the sweet emotions it elicits.

I would highly recommend this book to anyone walking through the NICU doors for the first time and to those that have spent years there."
—Krista Burrow Nuttall, Speech-language Pathologist, Neonatal Therapist

My NICU Story

www.ingramcontent.com/pod-product-compliance
Lightning Source LLC
LaVergne TN
LVHW041640070526
838199LV00052B/3471